The Diabetic Holy Grail

Your Guide to Learning

the Truth Behind Diabetes,

the Facts Behind the Myths

and 100% Stress Free Diet Plan

Christine Cawthorn

Digital Print House

Acknowledgments

I would like to recognize, acknowledge and applaud all the people around the world that helped make this book and this mission possible. I cannot name you all individually, but you know who you are. I am honored to serve with you on this noble mission of educating the world and helping each person becoming a better person today than yesterday.

Table of Contents

Introduction

You have diabetes. Perhaps this is a new discovery, perhaps not; regardless, the fact remains and you need to learn a new way of life. You have quickly discovered that countless people will offer advice, but no one really has the answers you need.

People tell you what they think they would do in your same situation, but their solutions for you are based on myths rather than fact.

Don't worry. I get it. I know what it's like to have people offer their best advice, but it leaves you feeling discouraged time and time again when it doesn't work. As you know, people may want to be helpful but it doesn't matter what their motives are when the solution doesn't do you any good.

I've wanted to write this book for a long time. My best friend was diagnosed with diabetes at a surprisingly young age, and I have stood by her with unending devotion, helping her regain the life she first dreamed she would have. It has been a journey that has had its ups and downs, but it hasn't been without its rewards.

Now I want to help you. This diagnosis is not your defining moment! I want to give you all the tidbits behind having diabetes, the truth of diet/exercise plans and how you can continue to enjoy the meals you have always loved with some creative variations suited for your new needs.

I want to show you that you can still live a normal life in spite of having diabetes. This book is going to change your life. In it, I am going to provide you with dozens of recipes you can enjoy. I am going to hand you your life back, and help you regain the carefree confidence you once had.

Don't wait. So much of life is wasted by waiting, and you have things to do!

I know so many secrets about the diabetic lifestyle you will never find on the internet. I can show you the things that only people who have learned through experience know, and I can teach you how to live the diabetic life worry-free. Not only are you going to feel better, but you are going to gain the confidence you need to boldly live life like you once did.

Here's to you living the rest of your life happier and healthier than ever.

Chapter 1

So You Have Diabetes

"The greater the obstacle, the more joy in overcoming it."

- Moliere

You have been diagnosed with a chronic disease that has left you staggering and wondering if you will ever get to enjoy life again. After all, when you think of someone who is battling any form of disease, all kinds of unpleasant thoughts come to mind. Fear begins to build.

How are you going to live the same kind of life? How are you going to enjoy things when you have to constantly check your blood sugar level? How are you supposed to relax and live life when you have the dread of a chronic illness hovering?

For many people, hearing that they have diabetes is shocking. Though they may acknowledge they haven't eaten right, realize they haven't exercised like they should or they know there is a history of diabetes in their family, they still never thought it was going to become a reality for them.

And you likely feel the same way.

If you look at diabetes from the outside, it's incredibly overwhelming. Suddenly, it does feel as though you aren't going to be able to do any of the things you once did or enjoy life in the same way. But, this isn't true.

In fact, many people who are given this diagnosis end up making changes in their lifestyle that make them feel better than ever in *spite of* having this disease. I want to get you to that point. I want you to be able to look back over your life and realize that once you made some of the changes you had to make, you are better than ever.

And to do that, I am going to start by giving you some of the facts behind diabetes, dispelling the myths behind the disease.

Myth: You get diabetes by eating sugar.

Fact: Sugar is not a direct cause of diabetes.

Type 2 diabetes is a result of a combination of factors, including genes, inactivity and overall lifestyle choices. Being overweight is a large contributing factor to developing Type 2 diabetes, and sugar may cause weight gain. But, in and of itself, sugar has no direct link to diabetes.

Myth: Type 2 diabetes doesn't require insulin.

Fact: Many cases of Type 2 diabetes requires insulin as the disease progresses.

Though people with Type 2 diabetes do not need to worry about injecting insulin when they are first diagnosed, there are plenty of cases in which the disease does require insulin later in life.

Right now, it's your goal to get this disease under control and managed through your diet and exercise regimen. Do what you can to avoid having to take insulin injections as you get older.

Myth: You have no warning and no control over a low blood sugar attack.

Fact: You can easily manage your symptoms through diet and exercise, and basically eliminate ever having to deal with any of these attacks.

In the past, people would often fear enjoying their daily activities because they may succumb to a blood sugar attack without warning. Fear was created because when your blood sugar gets too low, you may risk falling unconscious.

But, through proper diet and exercise, you can completely manage this disease and virtually eliminate the risk of ever having to face these attacks. Another thing to keep in mind is that you do have a warning when your sugar is dropping, and you do have time to take action before bad things occur.

It's not always convenient, but this isn't a disease that is going to control your life.

Myth: There's a way to cure diabetes.

Fact: Diabetes can be managed and potentially reversed through a variety of treatments and lifestyle choices, but there isn't a definite "cure" for the disease at this point.

If you look at the medical term for the word *"cure"*, it means that there is something you can do that will completely eliminate the disease.

For example: If you have strep throat, you go to the doctor. You are prescribed antibiotics. You take the pills as directed, and within a few days to a week, the illness is gone... it has been cured.

But, if you have cancer, you have to go in for various forms of treatment. Some of these treatments have been proven to reduce cancer, and for some patients, the cancer is eliminated, but the treatments don't always work for everyone, so while you can *treat* cancer, there is no *cure*.

The same applies to diabetes. You will see all over the internet that there are miracle cures that will get rid of the disease for good. But, the fact is... there is no cure. You can do plenty of things (and you *should* do these things) to manage and potentially reverse the disease, but there is no guarantee that what you do is going to completely eliminate the disease in your life.

But don't let this discourage you in any way!

I know hearing that you can't cure a disease you have is not the news you want. As we work our way through this book, you are going to see that you really can live life to the fullest in spite of the diabetes and still enjoy all the things you once did.

With over 200 million cases of diabetes affecting men, women and children around the globe, and nearly two million new cases diagnosed in the United States alone every year, this is an incredibly common condition.

The key to living the life you want to live (and the life you deserve to live) is having the facts. Once you dispel the myths, you have actual truth you can use to effectively change and live your life.

Next we'll dive into some of the concrete facts you need to get your life on track. In no time at all it will be as though you don't have the disease.

Chapter Takeaways

1. You are not alone; there are millions of diabetes cases worldwide, with over a million new cases arising every year in the U.S. alone.

2. With all the myths and assumptions that surround this disease, it can be hard to know what advice to take: learn to separate fact from fiction.

3. Stay positive and do what you have to do to manage this disease.

4. Diabetes is a disease that has no cure, but with the right attitude, diet and exercise, you can manage your life well for the best you possible.

5. Use the facts I have provided in this chapter to your advantage. Knowledge is an incredibly powerful thing and can change your life.

Chapter 2

What's Next?

"You don't have to see the entire staircase, just take the first step."

\- Martin Luther King, Jr.

I hope after reading the first chapter you are feeling encouraged, and are now ready to make some real and tangible changes to your life. The last takeaway in the prior chapter talks about knowledge. Knowledge isn't information. Information is helpful, but it's what you do with it in your own life that makes the real difference. Knowledge when you take the information and create real steps to change your life.

When it comes to a diabetes diagnoses, you likely feel lost and overwhelmed with all of the things you are supposed to do. Trust me, that is understandable. Again, don't worry. I have broken down everything you need to do make it work for you, no matter what a day looks like in your life.

As you know, you need to get on a new diet. Suddenly, carbs, sugars, and calories all matter... but you must not forget about nutrition or healthy activities.

When it comes to your new eating plan, you will be choosing the healthiest foods you can... meaning they are going to be packed with nutrients. Moderation is the key to any diet, and you need to learn how to limit the sugar and carb contents of what you are eating.

As I said in the last chapter, sugar didn't give you diabetes, *but,* sugar *does* directly affect your blood glucose. Carbs also hold a significant role in what is happening in your blood, so you have to know the levels of carbs you are consuming as well since that turns into sugars to fuel (and overwork) your diabetic body.

The most common goal all diabetics need to consider is how they will get to a healthy weight. It doesn't matter if you are five pounds or 500 pounds overweight, you have to get to the healthy weight range for your height and gender.

Along with losing weight and healthy eating comes calories in the foods you are eating, too. Let me be clear that you do not need to "get skinny" and you do not need to get a six pack or defined muscles all over your body. Healthy behaviors are the basis of the changes that will improve your life, and that's surprisingly not as difficult as you may think once you see all the opportunities!

In chapters five through seven, I am going to provide you with breakfast, lunch, dinner and even dessert options that are healthy but low in what you are trying to avoid. But understand your knowledge doesn't stop with healthy eating — you also need to find a workout pattern that's right for you.

I have no interest in recommending body builders exercises; I just want you to reach a healthy weight and get enough cardio to help your heart. The more you take care of your body now, the easier it's going to be for you to manage the disease or potentially reverse it later.

Most people agree that it's not exercise itself that they hate doing, it's the kind of exercise that leaves them feeling worn out (or that practically kills them). I don't want you to hate your workouts, so pick something you enjoy with enough variety that you want to keep learning and growing healthier.

All of this helps you get used to the numbers chart.

Many people who are living with diabetes want to regulate and reverse it through diet and exercise. But, many of these people also wonder how they are able to tell if what they are doing is working.

Of course some of the obvious things are going to show through right away as you improve your health. Clothes are going to fit differently. You will sleep better and you will feel better. You're going to see yourself losing weight.

But, that's not enough when it comes to managing an illness. You can't just base how you're doing at managing diabetes based on how you feel; you have to keep track of numbers.

From this point moving forward, when you are in the doctor's office you are going to be given a list of things to watch as well as a chart. But, I want to offer you more than that. I want to give you the numbers you need to watch daily, and show you how to track them over the long haul with the recipes I share.

First of all, you need to keep an eye on your blood sugar levels.

As a general rule of thumb, you want your blood sugar level to be around 70-130 mg/dL. This is standard for what your levels should be before a meal or around mid-afternoon.

Of course, when you eat your blood sugar is going to increase, especially depending on what you were eating. But, as a target, you want your blood sugar to still be beneath 180 mg/dL between one to two hours after a meal.

When you are about to engage in something physically demanding, such as exercising hiking, or doing anything that is going to require physical exertion, you should check your blood sugar, too, as working out burns energy (thus lowering the sugar available as energy to the body).

As a safe guard against dropping your blood sugar with a workout, make sure your level is at least 100 mg/dL before you start. If it's not, eat a small healthy snack then wait for half an hour or so before you exercise.

Naturally, at the end of the day, your blood sugar is going to reach a certain level and stay there as your body winds down for the night. In the evening, you are looking for a range between 100-140 mg/dL.

You may have noticed this is a little high, especially if you are on the upper end of the range, but that's fine. Your body is shutting down for the night, and everything is going to be handled entirely differently as you sleep and don't supply new sources of energy for your body throughout the night.

You also need to take blood pressure is also taken into consideration.

Diabetes affects your entire body, and it can make you more likely to have a heart attack or stroke because of how it acts on your different body systems.

Keeping an eye on your blood pressure is crucial for your health. The pressure your blood is putting on your arteries and heart as it is pumped through your body. There's a good middle ground as, just like your blood sugar reading, you don't want this too low or too high.

The top number, also known as the systolic number, is the pressure that is placed on your arteries when your heart is contracted. The bottom number, also known as the diastolic number, is the pressure that is placed on your arteries between beats.

For normal blood pressure, you want the top number to be between 90 and 120, and you want the lower number between 60 and 80. While you may find your blood pressure is high (especially if you have never really checked it routinely), there is good news: blood pressure is also managed easily through healthy diet and a good exercise routine.

The third part of the healthy triangle that important is weight.

Most people who are diagnosed with diabetes are overweight. It doesn't seem to really matter by how much, though it is common sense to realize that the heavier you are, the more strain you are putting on your body.

Healthy weight is always given in a range. There is no "one size fits all" when it comes to your weight, but there is a specific range for your age, gender and height.

For example: A 6-foot tall male is going to shoot for a weight range of 160-196 pounds, while a female at the same age who is 5 feet 5 inches tall will have a weight range of 117-130 pounds.

Know that there are other determining factors at play here. Muscle weighs more than fat, so if you are muscular, you are going to weigh more than a person who has little to no muscle.

Talk to your doctor about your weight range, as well as the other number ranges I have addressed in this chapter. You can learn a lot from keeping these numbers in a chart, but your doctor knows you personally. Remember you know yourself better than anyone else on the planet, so listen to your body as you work to get healthy and see just how much better you feel.

Chapter Takeaways

1. Learn to embrace the overall healthy diet plan of nutrient rich foods eaten in moderation. There's room to adjust and personalize your plan, but adopt it as a whole process for optimum health.

2. Find an exercise regimen that works for you and that you actually enjoy doing.

3. Get into the habit of checking your blood sugar level several times throughout the day, especially before doing something physically demanding as preventive tactics to improving your health.

4. Check your blood pressure level once a week and adjust your diet (and exercise) to get it down to a healthy range for your gender.

5. Learn your healthy weight range and set your goal to get your weight into this range.

Chapter 3

Deadly Diabetic Sins

"When you choose your actions, you choose your consequences."

- Dr. Phil

When you are diagnosed with anything, no matter what it is, you immediately feel the need to do whatever it is you aren't supposed to do. It is as though you feel the need to prove to both the world and yourself that you are able to do anything you want, even if that means you're going against what you're supposed to do.

When it comes to diabetes, it's true... you can do whatever you like. I can't tell you that there are things you can and can't do, but what I can tell you is this: do what you want and face the consequences. I don't want to give you a list of the foods you can't have, or you will be at the supermarket buying those very things.

There is a different way I want to approach this, both for your own good and for the health of your body. The reason I am going to do this differently than most is because I want you to know *why* you can't just have every little thing that comes to your mind.

When you have diabetes, you have to deal with things that are out of your control, which means you have to do good things for your own body. I want to take this opportunity now to show you the common mistakes many people make with their diet and exercise regiments, and how you can avoid doing those very things yourself.

First, I want to talk about the mistakes people make with their diets. There are a number of things that can go wrong when you are trying to follow any kind of diet, whether you are working on low carb and low sugar of if you are trying to manage your caloric intake.

When it comes to diabetes and you are trying to do all three, you are bound to run into a significant amount of issues along the way. But, don't worry. I am going to provide you with some of the most common mistakes a lot of diabetics make, and offer advice on how you can avoid making the same mistakes yourself.

So let's get started.

1. You avoid all carbs

When it comes to health and nutrition, not all foods are created equal. A carb is not simply a carb no matter what, and you do have to make an effort to watch what kinds of carbs you are eating.

Not all carbs are bad; it's the refined, white, processed carbs you want to watch. In other words, white pasta is something you want to avoid, but an apple is not. See the difference?

2. You focus too much on diet and "diabetic friendly" foods

Just because something is labeled *diet* or *diabetic friendly* doesn't mean that it is, and it's up to you to recognize what you will and won't put in your body.

Many times, these specialty foods make base requirements (such as being low in sugar or low carb), but they are far from healthy. My goal is to teach you how to use nutrition to your advantage. I don't want you to just avoid foods that are full of sugar and carbs, I want you to also choose foods that are rich in the nutrients you need.

3. You go too long without eating

Yes, we are all used to eating three times a day. I have promised that you will be able to live the life you are used to living, but that in itself requires a few changes.

For starters, you are going to have to eat regularly, and at more frequent intervals. Snack time is going to become the norm, and that's just the way things are going to have to be.

It's going to take some time, but it won't take long for you to get used to it. Once you are accustomed to the new normal, it's going to be second nature. After all, snacking doesn't have to be an event, just something you do in the morning and afternoon.

When it comes to settling into a diabetic lifestyle, or rather the kind of lifestyle you can use to reverse and manage your diabetes, you will have to get used to a few things, including reading nutrition information and introducing healthy snacking into your day.

It's not hard, it just requires that you take the time to do it. When you are used to eating on the run or just eating whatever junk you want whenever you feel like it, going to a regular schedule can feel out of place and strange. Trust me, as with anything else, you're going to get used to it in no time, and when that happens, the normal way of doing things is going to come as second nature.

And this is just half the battle. Let's take a second now to look at the common mistakes people make with exercising, and how you can avoid those.

1. You don't exercise enough

When it comes to diabetes, you want to lose weight. It's essential for your health, even if you aren't going to try to carve out a six pack abdomen. Many people start out enthusiastically, but as soon as the newness wears off, they are right back to where they started - or even worse than before they were diagnosed.

2. You exercise too much

I know this sounds funny to someone who is trying to lose weight, or to someone who has never exercised before and is trying to get into the swing of things, but trust me, it's possible to exercise too much.

You have to be careful on both ends of the spectrum, meaning you need to exercise enough, but you have to watch to ensure that you don't exercise too much, or you are going to run into problems on the other end.

3. You don't allow yourself to recover from a workout

This one sort of goes hand in hand with the second point. When you are working out and losing weight, you have to do it in moderation, just like everything else you do.

Of course you want to see the weight come off quickly and you want to feel better, look better and potentially reverse your diabetes. None of that is going to happen if you don't take care of your body along the way.

As I have said a few times already, it's important that you stick with your exercise regimen, and only add a few spins to it that suit your own particular situation.

I can promise you the results you hope to see are real, but it's up to you to make a change. Don't let the fact that it's hard or uncomfortable scare you. You can do anything you set your mind to, you just have to be determined to do it.

There's more to mistakes and setbacks people make when they are trying to settle into the diabetic lifestyle, but you always have to watch for things that are not on the list. Basically, you are going to do everything in moderation.

You can't plan out every single situation you will ever face, and there are going to be times when you have to figure out what you are going to do on the spot. But, with common sense and the right training, you can make an educated decision that is going to turn out better than what would have happened if you overreacted in one way or another.

To make this entire process easier, I have included a list of the 100 foods you should avoid as a diabetic. Largely, these foods are laden with sodium and sugars, but there are also foods that made the list simply because they are not good for you.

But beware. Just because you think a food falls into the realm of foods you can have by diabetic standards doesn't mean that the food is necessarily good for you, so I have included it in foods you need to avoid. It is my goal to give you a book that is going to change your life for the better, not push you into the realm of fake foods and labels.

So, read the list, and learn to shop for groceries accordingly. Of course, I have allowed for some foods occasionally, because there just are some foods you can't imagine not having every now and then. But, overall, stick to this list and you won't have an issue with your shopping.

Here are the top 100 foods you need to avoid as a diabetic.

- Processed grains (white flour)

- Sugary cereals (especially when they don't balance it with whole grains)

- White bread

- White pasta

- White rice

- French fries

- Fried tortillas (especially when made with white flour)

- Fried breaded chicken (when the breading is made with white flour)

- Canned veggies with added sodium

- Pickles (again with the sodium)

- Sauerkraut (sodium, sodium, sodium)

- Canned fruit with heavy syrup (sugars)

- Chewy fruit roll-up snacks

- Fruit snacks

- Premade pie crust

- Premade dessert cups

- Fruit juice popsicles

- Premade pizza dough

- Premade bread dough

- Premade pie filling

- Sweetened applesauce

- Sweetened fruit drinks

- Sweetened fruit and veggie blend drinks

- Soda

- Diet soda (may not have the sugar, but is incredibly bad for your health)

- Dried fruit

- Fatty cuts of meat (lean meat is fine)

- Full-fat dairy (2%, reduced fat, or light dairy is fine)

- Prepackaged baked goods (Hostess and Little Debbie are out)

- Coffee drinks (regular coffee is fine, but those syrups baristas use are loaded with sugar)

- Sausage and gravy (too fatty)

- Deep fried anything

- Minute-ready grains

- Ice cream

- Gelato (still high sugar content)

- Cookie batter from the tube

- Cinnamon rolls from the tube

- Pre-made pie crust

- Many premade pies (learn how to check the ingredients, or better yet, learn how to make your own)

- Wine (a surprising amount of sugar)

- Beer (there is a lot of carbs in beer)

- Mixed drinks (alcohol isn't the problem; sugar and carbs are)

- Normal cinnamon rolls (there are other healthier options)

- Battered and fried anything (again, with few exceptions)

- Processed lunch meats

- Processed pre-sliced cheese

- Fast food burgers

- Hot dogs (with few exceptions)

- Premade cookies

- Sweet teas

- Nachos

- Frozen dinners

- Frozen pizza

- Frozen breakfast sandwiches

- Fast food breakfast sandwiches

- Energy drinks

- Jams

- Jellies

- Prepackaged oatmeal

- Poptarts

- Donuts

- Bacon (except for on occasions if you really love bacon)

- Prepackaged chip dip

- Canned soups (watch the sodium, some exceptions may be ok)

- Frozen specialty desserts

- Movie theater popcorn (possibly fine, watch for the sodium)

- Popcicles

- Frozen appetizers

- Chips (except for the low sodium varieties)

- Syrups

- Chinese food

- Water flavor packets

- Water enhancement packets

- Low-quality salad dressings

- Prepackaged cake batter mixes

- Prepackaged baked mixes

- Candy (as a habit)

- Cake

- Restaurant desserts (with exceptions)

- Crackers (with exceptions)

- Food like products

- Excessive salt

- Coffee creamers (use sparingly, and watch out for sugars)
- "extra" anything (when you are ordering dinner, coffee, ice cream, etc.)
- Whipped cream
- Whipped topping (not the same as whipped cream)
- Frozen treats (other than ice cream)
- Cheez whiz
- Virtually anything that comes canned unless it's marked salt-free (sodium is a real issue here)
- Milk chocolate (a lot of sugar)
- Filled chocolates (more sugar)
- Chocolate liquors (sugar again)
- Premade glazes (and many homemade glazes)
- Premade coatings (especially candy coatings)
- Candied veggies
- Candied fruits
- Jerky (watch out for sodium here)
- Premade eggs (for scrambling)
- Premade frozen hamburger patties
- Added sugar to anything

As you read through this list, I'm sure you noticed two common factors through everything you saw. There are a lot of prepackaged items on the list and a lot of things that contain added sugar.

As you well know, you have to be really careful of added sugar and sodium, and when it comes to prepackaged foods, you are going to run into a lot of both. When you put a lot of salt into a food, you can preserve it for long periods of time. That's why when you are looking at the premade dinners and desserts, you will run into a lot of sodium, even if the finished product doesn't taste like salt.

I know when you first read this list it feels as though you have to let go of a lot of the foods you love. I want to show you that you can cook countless dinners at home that you can enjoy without worry. While it may seem like you have to avoid most of what is on the market today right now, you are going to quickly see that not only can you do better yourself, but you are going to prefer the food you can make at home over what you can buy frozen anyway.

Starting with the next chapter, I am going to show you countless recipes you can make and enjoy guilt free, worry free, and as you should.

Chapter Takeaways

1. Be careful not to become obsessed with what you can and can't have in your diet. Learn how to live and learn… there are going to be things you do and learn from, and other things you can do to avoid making a mistake.

2. Your exercise regimen is as important as your diet, and it requires that you put in the same effort and care to find what works for you.

3. Just like with your diet, it is possible to overdo… or underdo your exercise regimen. You have to find what works for you and works in general.

4. You have to keep an eye out for foods that are bad for you because of sugar, and because of carbs. Some may be one or the other, some may be both.

5. Sodium is also a culprit when it comes to diabetic issues. We don't see it addressed as much, but it is still something to watch, especially when you are dealing with high blood pressure.

Chapter 4

Thoroughly Breakfast

"Expect problems and eat them for breakfast"

- Alfred A. Montapert

As someone who has to be careful of what they eat, any food that falls restriction-free into the acceptable category is openly welcome. Here, I have put together a list of 26 breakfast recipes that you can enjoy without fear of what they may do to your diabetes or your day, so make each and every recipe, and fall in love with the results.

It's up to you and your doctor to decide how low you want to keep your carb intake, and these recipes are all for those who are aiming for a range of 50-90 grams per day. They are packed with nutrition, and none of these recipes will cause a major spike in your blood sugar.

Spinach Omelet Divine

Serves: 1 Carbs: 4g Sugars: 2g Calories: 235

What you will need:

1 cup spinach

2 eggs

Sprinkling of feta cheese

Pepper

Splash of 2% milk

Salt

Hot sauce

Drizzle of oil (for the pan)

Directions:

Whisk the eggs and milk together, then pour into a pan heated over medium heat with a little oil drizzled inside. Cook a few minutes, before adding spinach and cheese to the center.

Fold over and finish cooking, and enjoy!

Easy Broccoli Egg Bake

Serves: 1 Carbs: 7.7g Sugars: 2.4g Calories: 214

What you will need:

1 cup broccoli

2 eggs

Salt

Pepper

Tobacco sauce

Directions:

Whisk the eggs until smooth, then pour into a pan that has been preheated on the stove. Chop the broccoli and add to the mix, then cook with salt and pepper to taste.

Finish with a drizzle of the tobacco sauce, and enjoy!

Cottage Cheese Please

Serves: 1 Carbs: 8g Sugars: 8g Calories: 194

What you will need:

1 cup cottage cheese

Cinnamon

Directions:

Spoon the cottage cheese into a glass bowl and heat for about 30 seconds in the microwave. You want it to be warm, but not hot. Sprinkle some cinnamon on top, and enjoy!

Cocoa Parfait

Serves: 1 Carbs: 8.9g Sugars: 8.5g Calories: 200

What you will need:

1 cup cottage cheese

1 teaspoon baking cocoa

½ cup strawberries (fresh)

Directions:

Slice the strawberries and layer in a bowl with the cottage cheese and cocoa. Heat slightly, if desired, and enjoy!

Royal Strawberry Smoothie

Serves: 1 Carbs: 22 Sugars: 19g Calories: 175

What you will need:

1 cup low-fat milk

1 cup low-fat, plain yogurt

Splash of real vanilla

1 cup strawberries

Ice

Directions:

Blend all ingredients in your blender until smooth. Add the ice a little at a time until you get the consistency you want, and enjoy!

Cinnamon Cream of Wheat

Serves: Carbs: 27g Sugars: 6 Calories: 180

What you will need:

½ cup unsweetened vanilla almond milk

Cinnamon

1/3 cup cream of wheat cereal (unprepared)

Directions:

Prepare the cream of wheat with only water. Let set up for a few seconds, then pour ½ cup almond milk plus a sprinkling of cinnamon over the top and enjoy! (This should be about ¾ cup prepared)

Vanilla Smoothie Like No Other

Serves: 1 Carbs: 8g Sugars: 7g Calories: 80

What you will need:

1 cup unsweetened vanilla almond milk

Generous sprinkle of chia seeds

Vanilla

Directions:

The night before, combine your chia seeds, vanilla and almond milk. If you want it to be more pudding like in the morning rather than a drink, add more chia seeds. You really can't go wrong with these little power houses, and the result is simply delicious!

Muggy Eggs

Serves: 1 Carbs: 6g Sugars: 2g Calories: 160

What you will need:

2 eggs

Light sprinkling of salt

Pepper to taste

½ green pepper

Directions:

Chop the green pepper into bite sized pieces and beat together with your egg. Sprinkle a light bit of salt on top, then add pepper to taste. Pop in the microwave and let cook for 1 minutes, then open and stir and pop in for another minute.

Pull out and make sure it's fully cooked, then let stand for a minute and enjoy!

Egg Mash

Serves: 1 Carbs: 18g Sugars: 6.5g Calories: 200

What you will need:

2 eggs

½ cup broccoli

1 onion

½ cup cauliflower

Splash of almond milk

Salt and pepper to taste

Directions:

Chop all the ingredients as small as you can, and whisk with the eggs. Add in the splash of almond milk to ensure it's not too dry, then heat in a skillet on the stove over medium heat.

Stir often, and when done, serve immediately.

Cauliflower Fried Rice

Serves: 1 Carbs: 6.2g Sugars: 2g Calories: 176

What you will need:

2 eggs

Splash of plain, unsweetened almond milk

1 cup cauliflower

Salt and pepper to taste

Directions:

Heat a pan on the stove with a bit of olive oil, then chop the cauliflower as small as you can get it. Add the eggs and almond milk, then scramble on the stove until cooked through.

Let stand for a moment, and season with salt and pepper to taste. Enjoy!

Scrambled Egg Lettuce Wraps

Serves: 1 Carbs: 1.2 Sugars: 0.5g Calories: 190

What you will need:

2 eggs

Splash of low-fat milk

Salt and pepper to taste

Large leaf lettuce

Directions:

Whisk the milk with the eggs and cook slowly on a pan over medium heat. Once finished, season with salt and pepper to taste, then transfer to your large leaf lettuce.

Wrap and enjoy! You can also add a bit of your favorite dressing to the mix, but keep in mind this is going to add to the overall carb count.

Simple Stuffed Pepper

Serves: 1 Carbs: 12g Sugars: 4g Calories: 80

What you will need:

1 green pepper

1 cup green spinach

Feta cheese

Pepper to taste

Directions:

Cut open and wash out the green pepper, and chop the spinach. Preheat your oven to 350 degrees F.

Place the pepper in foil, and fill with spinach, then top with the feta cheese. Finish wrapping in foil, and place in the oven. Bake for 20 minutes, then season with the pepper to taste when done.

That's it! Enjoy!

Pepper Medley Saute

Serves: 1 Carbs: 28g Sugars: 8g Calories: 96

What you will need:

1 red pepper

1 green pepper

1 yellow pepper

1 orange pepper

Feta cheese

Directions:

Slice and clean all of the peppers, and make sure they are sliced thinly. Place on the stove heated over medium heat with a bit of olive oil.

Let cook until soft, garnish with feta, and enjoy right away.

Yogurt Egg Spinach Bake

Serves: 2 Carbs: 20g Sugars: 3g Calories: 200

What you will need:

4 eggs

1 cup spinach

1 cup plain, low fat yogurt

1 bunch green onions

Directions:

Chop the green onions, and place in a skillet on the stove. Heat over medium low heat, then add in the spinach, and stir in the yogurt. Finish by cracking the eggs in the center, and seasoning with light salt, pepper and garlic powder.

Cover and let bake on the stove for another 10 to 15 minutes. Enjoy!

Turkey Breakfast Skillet

Serves: 2 Carbs: 32.6g Sugars: 1.5g Calories: 587

What you will need:

1 pound turkey burger

Italian seasoning

2 eggs

Cilantro

Avocados

½ cup brown rice (cooked)

Directions:

Brown the turkey burger on the stove, and season with Italian seasoning and pepper to taste. Whisk the eggs together in a dish, then stir in with the turkey. Make sure you have ½ cup prepared brown rice, and add that in next, then season with the cilantro.

Slice the avocado, but keep this set aside for now. Continue to cook your skillet dish everything is well combined and cook through, then toss in the avocado and stir. Cook another 10 minutes, and serve.

Enjoy!

Turkey Bacon Wraps

Serves: 2 Carbs: 5.5g Sugars: 1.2g Calories: 388

What you will need:

1 package turkey bacon

4 eggs

Feta cheese

Pepper to taste

Directions:

Preheat your oven to 350 degrees F.

Wrap the bacon around the rings of 4 muffin sections in a muffin baking pan, greased lightly.

Crack the eggs and place 1 in each of the bacon rings. Garnish with feta cheese and pepper to taste.

Place in the oven and bake 20-25 minutes, until the bacon is done and the eggs are cooked. Enjoy!

Avocado Green Smoothie

Serves: 1 Carbs: 28g Sugars: 15g Calories: 334

What you will need:

1 avocado

1 tablespoon baking cocoa

Vanilla

Lemon juice

1 cup plain, low-fat yogurt

1/2 cup low-fat milk

Ice

Directions:

Slice the avocado into smaller pieces and remove the pit. Place in a blender with all other ingredients besides the ice. Turn on and blend well, then add the ice a little at a time until you are happy with the consistency of the smoothie.

Enjoy!

Pumpernickel Spread

Serves: 1 Carbs: 16g Sugars: 13g Calories: 150

What you will need:

1 slice pumpernickel bread

¼ cup plain, low fat yogurt

Cocoa powder

Vanilla

Directions:

In a bowl, combine the yogurt, cocoa powder and vanilla. Mix well, then spread evenly across the bread. Enjoy immediately.

7 Grains of Heaven

Serves: 1 Carbs: 27g Sugars: 3g Calories: 140

What you will need:

½ cup unsweetened vanilla almond milk

Splash of real vanilla

¼ cup 7 grain whole grain hot breakfast cereal

Cinnamon to taste

Directions:

Prepare the 7 grain cereal with water, according to the packaging directions. Once fully cooked, stir in the almond milk along with a splash of vanilla and sprinkle the cinnamon on top, to taste. Enjoy immediately.

Avocado Boats

Serves: 1 Carbs: 26g Sugars: 2g Calories: 367

What you will need:

1 avocado

2 eggs

Pepper

Hot sauce

Directions:

Slice the avocado in half lengthwise, and use your spoon to smash down the center (somewhat). Carefully crack the eggs, being careful not to break the yolk, and place in the center of the avocado halves.

Place in a bread pan or shallow baking dish and bake at 350 F for 20 minutes.

Season with pepper to taste, and garnish with hot sauce when you are ready to enjoy.

Cheater Muffins

Serves: 2 Carbs: 14.2g Sugars: 8.2g Calories: 324

What you will need:

2 cups cottage cheese

1 small bunch scallions

1 teaspoon chia seeds

1 tablespoon ground flax seeds

1 teaspoon baking powder

Pepper to taste

Feta cheese

3 eggs

Almond meal

Directions:

Preheat oven to 350 degrees F.

Chop the scallions and break 1 tablespoon feta cheese into much smaller pieces. Combine all ingredients except for the almond meal in a mixing bowl, then begin adding the almond meal until you have a muffin batter.

Line a muffin tin with liners, and pour the batter into the center. Bake in the oven for 30-40 minutes, until the muffins are a golden brown color.

Enjoy!

Delectable Pancakes

Serves: 1 Carbs: 9.2g Sugars: 2g Calories: 295

What you will need:

¼ brick lite cream cheese

2 eggs

Almond meal

Directions:

Heat a pan on the stove over medium heat. As this heats, soften your cream cheese and combine with the eggs. Add in the almond meal, a little at a time, until you have a pancake batter consistency (it will be thick).

Spoon 1/3 onto the pan and cook for 3 minutes, then flip and finish the other side.

Makes 3 medium pancakes. Enjoy!

Breakfast Salad

Serves: 1 Carbs: 32g Sugars: 4.2g Calories: 422

What you will need:

2 avocados

2 tomatoes

1 lemon

Salt to taste

Directions:

Slice the lemon and remove the skin and the seeds, then set aside. Chop the tomatoes and avocados, then combine everything in a dish, stirring gently, you don't want to break apart the tomatoes or smash the avocado.

Season with a bit of salt to your own taste, and enjoy!

Wheat Berries

Serves: 1 Carbs: 35g Sugars: 7.2g Calories: 170

What you will need:

1/3 cup whole wheat berries

Water

Vanilla

Cinnamon

Low-fat milk

Directions:

Cover the berries generously with water and let boil on the stove for close to an hour. You're going to know when they are done because they will be larger and soft.

Once the berries have finished cooking, remove from the heat and sprinkle cinnamon on top, along with a splash of vanilla and low-fat milk. Enjoy!

All About That Almond Smoothie

Serves: 1 Carbs: 10g Sugars: 7g Calories: 277

What you will need:

2 tablespoons almond butter

2 cups unsweetened vanilla almond milk

Chia seeds

2 tablespoons cocoa powder

Ice

Directions:

Combine all ingredients except for the ice in your blender and blend well. Be generous with the chia seeds; they are packed with protein! You may have to turn off the blender and scrape the almond butter off the side before you can continue.

Once blended, add in the ice a few cubes at a time, until you get the consistency you want. Enjoy!

Almond Butter Pumpernickel

Serves: 1 Carbs: 13g Sugars: 0.5g Calories: 247

What you will need:

1 slice pumpernickel bread

2 tablespoons unsweetened almond butter

Cinnamon

Vanilla

Directions:

Combine the almond butter, cinnamon, and vanilla in a bowl, then spread over your bread. Enjoy!

Chapter 5:

Thoroughly Lunch

"It's a good day to have a good day"

- Unknown

Breakfast takes all the glory as the most important meal of the day, but when it is important that you enjoy meals at regular intervals, no matter what their technical name is, you can't help but appreciate lunch for all that it does.

Now, take the stress out of your lunches and rest assured you are getting the most nutrition for your caloric dollar. Not only are these choices healthy, they are some of the most delicious lunch options you have ever enjoyed.

It's up to you and your doctor to decide how low you want to keep your carb intake, and these recipes are all for those who are aiming for a range of 50-90 grams per day. They are packed with nutrition, and none of these recipes will cause a major spike in your blood sugar.

Grilled Chicken Boats

Serves: 2 Carbs: 4g Sugars: 1g Calories: 153

What you will need:

2 chicken breasts

1 cup spinach

1 ball fresh mozzarella cheese

Pepper to taste

Fresh tomato

Olive oil

Directions:

Preheat oven to 350 degrees F.

Bake your chicken in the oven for 15 minutes, covered and with a bit of oil. As this bakes, slice the tomato and fresh mozzarella. Lay the cheese over the chicken, followed by the tomato and spinach, then place back in the oven for another 10 minutes.

Let sit out for a few minutes to cool, then enjoy!

Lettuce Wraps Deluxe

Serves: 1 Carbs: 2 Sugars: 0.5 Calories: 53

What you will need:

Chicken breast

Tomato

Large leaf lettuce

Favorite dressing

Directions:

Cut your chicken into bite sized pieces, and brown on the stove. You can use a bit of olive oil here if you like, but it's up to you. Lay out your lettuce, and chop your tomato.

Stuff everything inside the lettuce, and go light on your dressing (dressing does affect sugar and carb content, so plan accordingly).

Wrap up, and enjoy!

Roasted Delight

Serves: 1 Carbs: 19g Sugars: 8g Calories: 217

What you will need:

1 red onion

1 red pepper

5 asparagus stalks

1 cup mushrooms

1 cup chopped chicken

Directions:

Coarsely chop the veggies (or slice them if you would rather).

Lay out all ingredients on a baking sheet, and turn on the oven to 400 degrees F.

Drizzle with a bit of olive oil, and pop in the oven for 20 minutes, stirring halfway through. Once the chicken is done and the veggies are soft, you are ready to enjoy!

Cauliflower Fried Rice Lunch Style

Serves: 2 Carbs: 13.2g Sugars: 2g Calories: 435

What you will need:

2 eggs

1 chicken breast

1 green pepper

Splash of plain, unsweetened almond milk

1 cup cauliflower

Salt and pepper to taste

Directions:

Heat a pan on the stove with a bit of olive oil, then chop the cauliflower as small as you can get it. Add the eggs and almond milk, then scramble on the stove until cooked.

Chop the chicken and start browning on the stove in a separate dish. Once thoroughly cooked, add to the rest of the ingredients.

Let stand for a moment, and season with salt and pepper to taste. Enjoy!

Easy Tuna Salad

Serves: 1 Carbs: 5g Sugars: 5.5g Calories: 228

What you will need:

1 can tuna

1 cup spinach

Feta cheese

½ cup cherry tomatoes

Favorite low carb dressing

Directions:

Lay the spinach down on a plate, and open and drain the can of tuna. Spread this on next, then slice the tomatoes in half lengthwise and lay them down on top of the tuna.

Finish with the feta cheese as a garnish, and drizzle lightly with your favorite dressing.

Enjoy!

Easy Veggie Platter

Serves: 1 Carbs: 16.5g Sugars: 6.4g Calories: 232

What you will need:

2 boiled eggs

2 carrots, sliced

2 celery stalks, sliced

½ cup cherry tomatoes

Low-fat plain Greek yogurt

Garlic powder

Pepper, to taste

Directions:

Wash and slice the veggies into sticks, and cut the boiled eggs in half. Combine the yogurt and the garlic powder and pepper, to taste, then dip your veggies in the yogurt dip.

Enjoy!

Mozzarella Salad

Serves: 1 Carbs: 4.5g Sugars: 2g Calories: 330

What you will need:

1 small bunch green onions

1 ball fresh mozzarella cheese

1 can garbanzo beans

Garlic powder

Pepper to taste

Olive oil

Directions:

Chop the green onions into smaller pieces, and slice the mozzarella cheese in half first, then into strips. Combine in a dish. Open and drain the can of chickpeas, then rinse under water to eliminate excess sodium.

Add half the can to the mix, save the other half for another day. Season with garlic powder and pepper to taste, then drizzle a small amount of olive oil over the top.

Serve immediately.

Delectable Egg Salad

Serves: 1 Carbs: 42g Sugars: 7g Calories: 352

What you will need:

1/3 cup chickpeas

2 boiled eggs

1 teaspoon mayo

1 teaspoon mustard

Dill seasoning

Garlic seasoning

Pepper to taste

Directions:

Open and drain the can of chickpeas, then rinse under cold water to get rid of the excess sodium. Smash the eggs with a fork, and combine all ingredients in a dish.

Make sure all are thoroughly combined and season to your personal taste. Serve with low carb veggies of choice.

Best Ever Personal Pizza

Serves: 1 Carbs: 34g Sugars: 7g Calories: 252

What you will need:

1 Whole wheat (or whole grain) English muffin

1 can tomato paste

Fresh mozzarella

Fresh tomato

Avocado

Directions:

Cut the English muffin in half and spread the tomato paste on top. Chop the fresh tomato (I prefer Romas) and slice the mozzarella. Cut the avocado in half and smash this as well.

Add the avocado next, then lay the cheese on top of that. Sprinkle the tomato on top, and pop in the oven preheated to 350 degrees F. for 20 minutes.

Serve immediately.

Mini Salmon Sandwich

Serves: 1 Carbs: 30g Sugars: 4g Calories: 545

What you will need:

1 frozen salmon patty

1 whole wheat or whole grain English muffin

Roma tomato

Lemon juice

Directions:

Cook the salmon over medium heat on the stove, and garnish with a bit of lemon juice. As the salmon cooks, wash the arugula, and slice the tomato. Toast the English muffin, and once the salmon is finished cooking, assemble your sandwich.

Serve immediately.

Hummus Avocado Toast

Serves: 1 Carbs: 32g Sugars: 2g Calories: 180

What you will need:

1 slice whole grain bread (or any low carb variety of your choice)

3 tablespoons hummus

½ avocado

Pepper to taste

Directions:

Smash the avocado, and toast your whole grain bread. Spread the hummus over the toast, then spread the avocado on top of that.

Season with pepper, to taste.

Enjoy!

Diabetic Approved Cheesy Pasta

Serves: 1 Carbs: 47g Sugars: 6.1g Calories: 417

What you will need:

1 cup prepared 100% whole wheat pasta

½ cup cherry tomatoes

Mozzarella cheese

¼ cup chickpeas

Olive oil

Directions:

Prepare the pasta according to the packaging directions, but leave out the salt. Slice the cherry tomatoes and mozzarella cheese, then open and drain the can of chickpeas.

Rinse the chickpeas to get rid of any excess sodium, then combine everything in a dish.

Drizzle a bit of olive oil over the top, and enjoy.

Cheater Mac 'n' Cheese

Serves: 1 Carbs: 18g Sugars: 10g Calories: 587

What you will need:

1 cup cheddar cheese

½ cup cottage cheese

Mustard

1 cup cauliflower

½ cup low-fat milk

Pepper to taste

Directions:

Melt the cheeses with the milk over medium heat on the stove. Chop the cauliflower, but not too small. Combine with the cheese, and stir.

Add in the pepper to taste, as well as a squirt of mustard.

Enjoy immediately.

Heavenly Diabetic Grilled Cheese

Serves: 1 Carbs: 40g Sugars: 4g Calories: 197

What you will need:

½ cup cottage cheese

1 whole wheat English muffin

2 teaspoons coconut oil

Pepper to taste

Directions:

Preheat a pan on the stove over medium heat. Spread the coconut oil across both slices of muffin, and place on the pan.

Spread the cottage cheese on next, carefully so you don't burn yourself, and garnish with pepper to taste.

Cook on one side for 3 minutes, then flip over and continue to cook on the other side for another 3 minutes, until cooked thoroughly.

Enjoy immediately.

Apples to Oranges

Serves: 1 Carbs: 42g Sugars: 26g Calories: 212

What you will need:

1 apple

1 orange

2 tablespoons almond butter

Directions:

Slice the orange and the apple, and spread the almond butter over the apple slices. Enjoy!

Salmon Tacos

Serves: 1 Carbs: 28g Sugars: 1g Calories: 529

What you will need:

1/3 pound cooked salmon

2 corn tortillas

Green onion

Lime juice

Cilantro

Plain, low-fat Greek yogurt

Directions:

Cook your salmon then shred it and heat the corn tortillas in the microwave. Chop the green onion, and combine everything as a taco.

Use the lime juice as a garnish, and enjoy immediately.

Grapefruit Salad

Serves: Carbs: 20g Sugars: 8g Calories: 232

What you will need:

1 grapefruit

1 handful spinach

1 handful romaine

4 regular sized shrimp, cooked

Drizzle low carb dressing of your choice

Directions:

Wash the leaves and remove the tails from the cooked shrimp. Slice the grapefruit and remove from its skin, then assemble.

Top with low carb dressing of choice, and serve immediately.

Specialty Peppers

Serves: 1 Carbs: 11g Sugars: 2.4g Calories: 517

What you will need:

1 egg

¼ brick cream cheese

2 green onions

1 red pepper

Cheddar cheese

Cilantro

Directions:

Core the pepper and remove the seeds, then soften the cream cheese in the microwave. Chop the green peppers, and combine with the cream cheese, then stuff in the middle of the pepper. Add the egg next, carefully so you don't break the yolk.

Top with cheddar cheese, and bake in the oven at 350 degrees F for 20-30 minutes. Serve immediately.

Low Carb Stir Fry

Serves: 1 Carbs: 19g Sugars: 13g Calories: 127

What you will need:

1 cup mushrooms

1/3 cup broccoli

¼ cup cauliflower

Shredded carrots

Olive oil

Feta cheese

Directions:

Combine all the ingredients except for the feta in a pan turned on to medium heat. Sauté in olive oil, and remove from heat when the veggies are thoroughly cooked.

Garnish with the feta cheese, and you are done.

Enjoy immediately.

Broccoli Cheese Sleaze

Serves: 1 Carbs: 13g Sugars: 5g Calories: 504

What you will need:

1 cup broccoli

1 cup shredded cheddar cheese

1 green pepper

Pepper to taste

Coconut oil

Directions:

Slice and wash the green pepper, and cut the broccoli into smaller pieces. Combine both in a pan on the stove with a little bit of coconut oil, then sprinkle the cheese on top.

Let the cheese melt as the veggies cook, and enjoy immediately.

World's Best Cheeseburger

Serves: 1 Carbs: 11g Sugars: 4g Calories: 422

What you will need:

Roma tomato

Cheddar cheese

¼ pound turkey burger

Salt and pepper to taste

Dill seasoning

Large leaf lettuce

1 tablespoon mayonnaise

Directions:

Brown the burger on the stove with the salt and pepper added to taste, then add a bit of the dill seasoning for the pickle flavor.

Add a slice of cheddar cheese on top, and lay out the lettuce on a plate. Spread the mayo on next, and layer everything on the lettuce.

Enjoy.

Hamburger Skillet

Serves: 1 Carbs: 9g Sugars: 3g Calories: 297

What you will need:

1/3 pound turkey burger

1 cup broccoli

½ cup cauliflower

1 egg

Salt and pepper to taste

Directions:

Chop the veggies and start the burger on the stove with the egg mixed in. Season with salt and pepper to taste, then, once the burger is about halfway done, add in the veggies.

Let finish cooking together, stirring often. Serve immediately.

Chocolate Almond Butter Lunch Smoothie

Serves: 1 Carbs: 26g Sugars: 13g Calories: 318

What you will need:

2 tablespoons almond butter

1 avocado

2 cups low fat milk

2 tablespoons cocoa powder

Vanilla

Ice

Directions:

Cut the avocado into smaller pieces, and remove the pit. Place in the blender with all the other ingredients except for the ice.

Turn on the blender and blend well, then begin adding in the ice cubes, a few at a time until you get the desired consistency.

Serve immediately.

Little Dippers

Serves: Carbs: 39g Sugars: 25g Calories: 292

What you will need:

1 large apple

1/3 cup semi-sweet chocolate chips

1 tablespoon almond butter

Directions:

Slice the apple into normal slices, and melt the chocolate chips with the almond butter on the stove. You can add a bit of almond milk or low-fat milk if you like, but this isn't necessary.

Once melted, remove from the heat and serve with the apple.

Enjoy immediately.

Diabetic Cream of Soup

Serves: 1 Carbs: 10.5g Sugars: 0.5g Calories: 200

What you will need:

1 can low sodium cream of mushroom soup

1 cup fresh mushrooms

Swiss cheese to garnish

Directions:

Heat the soup on the stovetop over medium heat. Season with pepper, to taste, if desired. Add in the fresh mushrooms, and let cook.

Once all is heated, garnish with a bit of the shredded Swiss cheese.

Enjoy!

Diabetic PB and J

Serves: 1 Carbs: 42g Sugars: 4g Calories: 398

What you will need:

Whole wheat English Muffin

1 tablespoon sugar free jam or jelly

2 tablespoons almond butter

Directions:

Assemble as you would any good ole' jelly and butter sandwich. Enjoy!

Your Fave Chicken and Noodles

Serves: 1 Carbs: 42g Sugars: 2g Calories: 426

What you will need:

1 boneless skinless chicken breast

1 celery stalk

1 cup prepared whole wheat pasta

Pepper to taste

Olive oil

Directions:

Cut the chicken into bite sized pieces and brown in a bit of olive oil on the stove. Slice the celery and add this to the mix.

As the celery and chicken cook, prepare the pasta according to the packaging directions, without the salt.

Combine everything, and enjoy!

Chapter 6

Thoroughly Dinner

"All great change… begins at the dinner table"

- Ronald Reagan

Dinner is one of two things… for starters, it is the biggest meal of the day. It takes the most time to prepare, it's often looked forward to the most and it's the biggest meal you are going to enjoy if you are counting calories.

It is also the cap of the day, bringing together families or couples. Dinner is simply something you look forward to because it means the hassles of the day are over. Regardless of what dinner means to you, these are the best dinner recipes to keep on hand if you are concerned about calories, carbs or sugars.

Make up any or all of these recipes without worry of what is inside… they are packed with nutrition and full of good things both inside and out.

It's up to you and your doctor to decide how low you want to keep your carb intake, and these recipes are all for those who are aiming for a range of 50-90 grams per day. They are packed with nutrition, and none of these recipes will cause a major spike in your blood sugar.

Elegant Chicken Enchiladas

Serves: 6 Carbs: 24g Sugars: 8g Calories: 417

What you will need:

1 pound boneless skinless chicken breast

1 green pepper

Corn tortillas

Mild salsa

1/3 cup plain, low-fat Greek yogurt

Directions:

Cut the chicken into bite sized pieces and brown on the stove in a bit of olive oil. Meanwhile, warm the tortillas in the microwave, and wash then chop the green pepper. Combine the green pepper and 1 cup of the salsa in a bowl, and season with cumin and cayenne pepper to taste.

Spread the yogurt across the tortillas, then finish with the toppings. Make sure the chicken is fully cooked before adding to the enchiladas.

Bake in the oven at 350 degrees F. for 10-15 minutes, and enjoy!

Salmon Salad Divine

Serves: 2 Carbs: 41g Sugars: 3g Calories: 589

What you will need:

1 pound fresh salmon

2 cups spinach

Lemon juice

1/2 cup prepared wheat berries

Feta cheese

Directions:

Cook the salmon on the stove over medium heat until it's completely cooked. Sprinkle a bit of lemon juice over the top, and set aside.

Wash and lay out the spinach, then sprinkle the wheat berries on top, ½ cup per plate. Lay the salmon on top of this bed you have made, then garnish with the feta cheese.

Finish with another spritz of lemon juice, and enjoy!

Super Salsa

Serves: 2 Carbs: 47g Sugars: 4g Calories: 764

What you will need:

1/3 cup black beans (rinse off the beans if you use canned)

1 can green chili peppers

1 can olives (rinse off)

¼ cup fresh frozen corn

1 can diced tomatoes (low sodium)

2 boneless skinless chicken breasts

Directions:

Open the cans and drain off the liquid. For all of these canned foods, rinse them off to get all of the extra sodium off of them.

Prepare the corn according to the packaging directions, and bake the chicken in the oven until cooked through.

Place the chicken on your plate first, then combine all other ingredients and spoon over the chicken breast.

Enjoy!

Shepherd's Pie Done Right

Serves: 4 Carbs: 32g Sugars: 3g Calories: 237

What you will need:

1 pound turkey burger

1 large bag frozen green beans

3 cups cauliflower

1 cup low-fat milk

1 jar tomato sauce (low sugar or sugar free, if possible)

Directions:

Press the turkey burger on the bottom of a 9x13 inch baking dish. Season with salt and pepper to taste. Prepare the green beans according to the packaging directions, and place them in the pan next.

Make cauliflower mashed potatoes by combining the cauliflower, egg, and milk in your blender, and while this blends add the tomato sauce to your mix in the pan.

Frost with the cauliflower, and season with paprika to taste.

Place in the oven at 350 degrees F. for 45 minutes.

Enjoy immediately.

Zucchini Boats

Serves: 2 Carbs: 12g Sugars: 4g Calories: 366

What you will need:

3 eggs

1 can tuna

1 large zucchini

Feta cheese

Salt and pepper to taste

Directions:

Cut open the zucchini and scoop out the center. Slice this smaller and add to a dish. Open and drain the can of tuna and mix with the zucchini, then add in the eggs. Season with salt and pepper to taste, and place in the oven on a baking sheet.

Bake at 350 degrees F for 45 minutes, then garnish with the feta cheese. Place back in the oven and bake for an additional 10 minutes, then serve.

Salmon Burgers

Serves: 1 Carbs: 16.5g Sugars: 4g Calories: 568

What you will need:

1 egg

1 green onion

1 slice English Muffin

1 small can salmon

Salt and pepper to taste

Directions:

Open and drain the can of salmon, chop the green onion and tear up the bread into small pieces. Combine everything in a mixing bowl, and heat a little bit of olive oil in a pan on the stove.

Form patties out of the salmon mix, and cook on the stove for 3 minutes on each side, or until you know the eggs have been cooked entirely.

Serve with hot sauce.

Wild Rice Spinach Skillet

Serves: 1 Carbs: 41g Sugars: 3g Calories: 322

What you will need:

1/4 cup prepared wild rice

1/4 cup black beans

1 cup spinach

1 can cream of mushroom soup (low sodium)

Pepper to taste

Directions:

If you are using canned beans, make sure you rinse them off to get rid of the excess sodium. Open the can of cream of mushroom soup, and combine the soup with the prepared wild rice and black beans.

Heat in a skillet on the stove over medium heat, and once heated through, add in the spinach. Season with pepper to taste, and let cook for 10 minutes.

Serve immediately.

Homemade Tomato Soup

Serves: 3 Carbs: 27g Sugars: 4g Calories: 389

What you will need:

3 cans diced tomatoes (low sodium)

¼ cup black beans

1 cup low-fat milk

Basil

Pepper to taste

Directions:

Place the tomatoes in a blender and blend on high to break up the pieces as small as you can. Open and drain the black beans, and rinse them off to ensure you get rid of the excess sodium.

Combine all ingredients in a pan on the stove, and heat over medium heat. Season to taste, and once heated through, serve immediately.

Garnish with cheddar cheese, if desired.

Wheat Berry Salad

Serves: 1 Carbs: 36g Sugars: 4g Calories: 315

What you will need:

1 can tuna

1/4 cup prepared wheat berries

1 can olives

1 green onion

Directions:

Open and drain the can of tuna, and open and drain the can of olives. Rinse the olives in cold water to rinse of excess sodium, and heat the wheat berries on the stove. Make sure you end up with 1/4 cup of prepared wheat berries.

Slice the olives into smaller pieces, and chop the onion.

Combine all ingredients and heat through, then serve.

Scrambled Egg Munch

Serves: 2 Carbs: 9g Sugars: 4g Calories: 273

What you will need:

½ pound turkey breakfast sausage

4 eggs

½ cup fresh mushrooms

Splash of low-fat milk

Pepper to taste

Directions:

Whisk the eggs with the milk and slice the mushrooms. Cook the sausage on the stove, and combine all ingredients in another pan. Cook over medium heat, and serve immediately.

Cowboy Beans

Serves: 2 Carbs: 32g Sugars: 4g Calories: 332

What you will need:

1/4 cup pinto beans

1/4 cup black beans

1/4 can baked beans

1 pound turkey sausage

Directions:

Open and rinse the cans of pinto beans and black beans to get rid of the excess sodium. Cook the turkey burger in a pan on the stove, and season with pepper to taste.

Open the can of baked beans and combine with the turkey burger, then add in the rest of the beans. Let heat completely through, and serve immediately.

Pork and Beans

Serves: 1 Carbs: 20g Sugars: 0.5g Calories: 311

What you will need:

1 pork chop

1/3 cup pinto beans

Ketchup

Directions:

Cook your pork chop thoroughly, making sure it's completely cooked. Remove from the bone, and cut into bite sized pieces. Open and rinse the can of pinto beans, then place in the pan with the pork chop.

Add a bit of ketchup to create a sauce, and mix well. Once heated through, serve immediately.

Easy Chicken Salad Sandwich

Serves: Carbs: 5g Sugars: 4g Calories: 350

What you will need:

1 boneless skinless chicken breast

1 large leaf lettuce

½ cup shredded cucumber

3 tablespoons light mayo

Olive oil

Directions:

Cook the chicken thoroughly, and cut into small pieces (smaller than bite sized). Stir the mayo and some olive oil in with the shredded cucumber, and stir in the chicken.

Transfer everything to your lettuce, and wrap.

Enjoy immediately.

Sweetness and Sours

Serves: 1 Carbs: 52g Sugars: 8g Calories: 388

What you will need:

1 cup fresh pineapple

1 pork chop

1 can cream of celery soup (low sodium)

1/4 cup prepared wild rice

Directions:

Cut the pork chop off the bone and into bite sized pieces. Cook thoroughly, then open and add the can of soup. Add a splash of low-fat milk, if desired.

As this heats, prepare the wild rice according to the packaging. Make sure you end up with 1 cup of wild rice prepared. Stir the pineapple in with the mix, and serve on top of the wild rice.

Enjoy immediately.

Cream of Celery Soup

Serves: Carbs: 18g Sugars: 6g Calories: 320

What you will need:

1 cup low-fat milk

4 celery stalks

1 can cream of celery soup (low sodium)

1 green onion

Directions:

Mince the celery and heat on the stove with the milk. Once heated, open and can of cream of celery soup and add to the mix. Chop the onion, coarsely. Add this to the mix, and let the soup simmer for 20 minutes.

Use a stick blender to smooth the soup, and enjoy.

Corn Chowder

Serves: 2 Carbs: 65g Sugars: 4g Calories: 465

What you will need:

½ cup frozen corn

1 cup low-fat milk

Salt and pepper to taste

1 cup chopped onion

1 potato

Directions:

Heat the corn according to the packaging directions, and add to a pot with the milk and chopped onion. Heat, and as it heats, peel and mince the potato, then add to the mix.

Season with salt and pepper, and once the soup has simmered for a few minutes, use your immersion (stick) blender to pureé well.

Serve immediately.

Pork Chop Salad

Serves: 2 Carbs: 41g Sugars: 18g Calories: 267

What you will need:

2 pork chops

1 small head cabbage

1 onion

Vegetable oil

Vinegar

Mustard

Celery seasoning

Pepper to taste

Directions:

Shred the cabbage and cut the pork chops off the bone. Cook the pork chops thoroughly. As they cook, combine 4 tablespoons vegetable oil with ½ cup vinegar and a squirt of mustard.

Add celery salt to this dressing, and pepper to taste. Mix well. Cut the pork chops into bite sized pieces, and toss everything together in a large salad bowl.

Let chill overnight and through the next day, then enjoy!

Cauliflower Tuna Melt

Serves: 1 Carbs: 5.5g Sugars: 5g Calories: 597

What you will need:

1 can tuna

1 cup cauliflower

½ cup shredded cheese

Salt and pepper to taste

Directions:

Open and drain the can of tuna, and wash the cauliflower. Combine in a pan and add salt and pepper, then heat for a few minutes, until the cauliflower is nearly done.

Add the cheese and let melt, then serve immediately.

Cabbage Soup

Serves: 2 Carbs: 36g Sugars: 5g Calories: 189

What you will need:

½ head cabbage

3 carrots

1 can diced tomato (low sodium)

Salt and pepper to taste

Onion

Water

Directions:

Chop all the veggies as coarsely or as finely as you want, and open the can of diced tomatoes. Combine everything in a pot on the stove and cover generously with water.

Bring to a boil then turn down to let simmer, and let simmer for an hour. Serve immediately.

Arugula Salad

Serves: 1 Carbs: 39g Sugars: 4g Calories: 655

What you will need:

1 cup arugula

1/3 cup cheddar cheese

¼ cup chickpeas

1/3 diced red onion

Directions:

Cube the cheese and open and rinse the can of chickpeas. Dab the chickpeas with a towel to dry them, and combine all ingredients in a mixing bowl.

Season with salt and pepper and a bit of olive oil, and serve.

Three Bean Slaw

Serves: 1 Carbs: 28g Sugars: 4g Calories: 451

What you will need:

1/3 cup green beans

1/3 cup great northern beans

1/3 cup pinto beans

1 carrot, shredded

1 can tomato paste

Pepper to taste

Directions:

If you are using canned beans, make sure you drain them and rinse them with cold water before using them. Combine with the tomato paste and shredded carrot, adding a little water if the paste is too thick.

Heat in a pan on the stove until heated through, and serve immediately.

Carrot Raisin Salad

Serves: 1 Carbs: 39g Sugars: 26g Calories: 156

What you will need:

2 carrots

1/3 cup raisins

Splash of low-fat milk

¼ cup plain, low-fat Greek yogurt

Pepper to taste

Directions:

Shred the carrots and combine with the raisins. In a separate bowl, combine the rest of the ingredients, then combine all ingredients. Serve.

Low Carb Chicken Dippers

Serves: 2 Carbs: 24g Sugars: 2g Calories: 460

What you will need:

2 boneless skinless chicken breasts

1 egg

Almond meal

Salt and pepper to taste

Dipping sauce of choice

Directions:

Preheat oven to 350 degrees F.

Crack the egg in a bowl, and slice the breasts into thick strips. Dip these first into the egg, then roll in the almond meal. Finish with salt and pepper to taste, and place on a cookie sheet.

Bake in the oven for 30 minutes, then flip over and bake an additional 30 minutes.

Let stand for a moment on a hot pad, then dip in your favorite sauce.

Low Carb French Toast

Serves: Carbs: 36g Sugars: 4g Calories: 212

What you will need:

English Muffin

Egg

Splash of low fat milk

Cinnamon

Directions:

Heat a pan over medium heat on the stove, and combine the egg with the bit of milk. Dip the English muffin in this mix, then place in the pan on the stove.

Sprinkle with cinnamon, and cook for 3 minutes on each side, until the eggs are cooked thoroughly.

Serve immediately with serving of choice.

Best Ever Shredded Pork Salad

Serves: Carbs: 22g Sugars: 5g Calories: 336

What you will need:

1 bag frozen peas

1 pork chop

2 tablespoons mayo

1 teaspoon dill seasoning

Pepper to taste

Directions:

Cook the pork chop thoroughly, then use your fork to shred the meat. Once shredded, combine with the mayo, pepper and dill seasoning. Meanwhile, cook the peas according to the packaging directions, then gently mix this in with the shredded meat.

Enjoy with a whole wheat English muffin, or the dipping tool of your choice… even great just eaten with a fork!

Zucchini Bake

Serves: Carbs: 21g Sugars: 15g Calories: 462

What you will need:

1 jar tomato sauce (no sugar added, low sodium)

1 yellow zucchini

1 green zucchini

1 pound turkey burger

Mozzarella cheese

1 cup cottage cheese

Directions:

Slice the zucchini lengthwise, and lay a bottom layer in a baking pan. Brown the turkey burger while you are doing this, and season with burger with pepper to taste.

Next, spread a layer of tomato sauce over the zucchini, then some burger. Add more zucchini next, then cottage cheese, followed by another layer of zucchini.

Finish the tomato sauce and burger next, then sprinkle shredded mozzarella cheese over the top.

Pop in the oven at 350 degrees F to bake for 45 minutes.

Serve immediately.

Chapter 7

Heavenly Desserts

"A party without a cake is just a meeting"

- Julia Child

Let's face it. We all love a nice breakfast, a good lunch sets the tone for the afternoon; you just can't beat a fancy dinner. Even the plain and simple dinners take the cake when they are well done, and you pride yourself in all the ways you are able to liven up the simplest of ingredients.

But, when it comes to dessert, there's just no substitute. You want chocolate. You want fruit. You want glazes and sweets. You want cakes and pies and ice creams. When it comes to dessert, there's just no second-best.

Don't worry. There are a number of desserts out there that are well within your range of acceptable foods, and I have little doubt you are going to fall in love with each and every dessert I have listed here.

Diabetes is nothing when you have a good cookbook in hand, and that's what I aim to provide you with here. So go ahead and have a slice of cake.

It's up to you and your doctor to decide how low you want to keep your carb intake, and these recipes are all for those who are aiming for a range of 50-90 grams per day. They are packed with nutrition, and none of these recipes will cause a major spike in your blood sugar.

Delightful Truffles

Serves: 12 Carbs: 5g Sugars: 3g Calories: 64

What you will need:

½ cup chocolate chips

½ cup almond butter

1/3 cup crushed peanuts

Directions:

Melt the chocolate chips over medium heat, and roll the peanuts inside the almond butter.

Form into balls, then use a fork to dip them into the melted chocolate. Set on waxed paper to set up, and enjoy!

Honeycombs

Serves: 24 Carbs: 7g Sugars: 4g Calories: 63

What you will need:

½ cup butter

2/3 cup honey

Whole wheat pastry dough

Vanilla

1 egg

Salt to taste

Directions:

Preheat oven to 350 degrees, and in a separate mixing bowl combine all ingredients. Mix well; you're going to have to work at it to get the ingredients mixed in with the dough.

Use a rolling pin to spread the dough out, and use cookie cutters to give it the honeycomb shape.

Place in the oven and bake for 8-10 minutes. Enjoy!

Frozen Tails

Serves: 1 Carbs: 19g Sugars: 22g Calories: 144

What you will need:

½ cup chocolate chips

1 banana

Directions:

Melt the chocolate chips and dip the banana inside. Lay on parchment paper in your freezer until frozen, then enjoy!

Devilishly Good Strawberries

Serves: 2 Carbs: 20g Sugars: 14g Calories: 133

What you will need:

½ cup dark chocolate chips

6 strawberries

Directions:

Melt the chocolate chips over medium heat on the stove, and wash the strawberries. Dip the strawberries about halfway into the chocolate, then let dry on parchment paper.

Enjoy!

Chia Pudding

Serves: 1 Carbs: 18g Sugars: 17g Calories: 115

What you will need:

1/3 cup chia seeds

1 cup chocolate almond milk

Directions:

Combine and leave in the fridge for 24 hours. Enjoy!

Fudgey Brownie Delight

Serves: 4 Carbs: 24g Sugars: 15g Calories: 142

What you will need:

1 ½ cup almond flour

¾ cup Splenda

2 tablespoons molasses

Salt to taste

½ cup plain, unsweetened almond milk

1 egg

1 cup canola oil

1 cup strong coffee

¼ cup cocoa powder

2 teaspoons baking powder

Directions:

Preheat oven to 350 degrees F.

In a mixing bowl, combine all ingredients, then transfer to a greased baking pan.

Bake in the oven for 20-30 minutes, testing with a butter knife to ensure it's done before you take it out of the oven. Enjoy!

Pumpkin Spice

Serves: 1 Carbs: 9g Sugars: 4g Calories: 45

What you will need:

1 packet Splenda

Splash of vanilla

1 cup pumpkin puree

Cinnamon

Nutmeg

Directions:

Start with blending the pumpkin and the vanilla, then add in the Splenda. From there, add in the spices, as many as you would like for your own personal taste.

Chill for half an hour, then enjoy!

Also good served hot.

Delicious Sugar Deluxe

Serves: 18 Carbs: 8g Sugars: 3g Calories: 54

What you will need:

1 ½ cups almond flour

Salt to taste

½ cup baking Splenda

2 tablespoons butter

2 tablespoons coconut oil

2 teaspoons real vanilla

1 egg

1 teaspoon baking powder

Cinnamon

Directions:

Preheat oven to 350 degrees F.

Mix ingredients in the order they are given, mixing thoroughly between each one. When you have a nice dough, grease a cookie sheet, then roll the cookies into 2 inch balls between your palms.

Press down lightly on the cookie sheet, then bake 8-10 minutes on the top rack of your oven. Let cool before you enjoy.

Peaches 'n' Cream

Serves: 1 Carbs: 14g Sugars: 13g Calories: 99

What you will need:

1 peach

1 packet Splenda

1/3 cup cream

Directions:

Slice your peach and lay it out prettily on a plate. Mix the Splenda with the cream, then pour over the peach. Enjoy!

Delectable Blueberry Parfait

Serves: 1 Carbs: 31g Sugars: 28g Calories: 144

What you will need:

1 /3 cup plain Greek yogurt

1 cup blueberries

1 packet Splenda

½ cup chocolate chips

Directions:

Combine Splenda with yogurt, then layer all ingredients in a dessert dish. Layer according to your own preference, and enjoy!

Heavenly Chocolate Cake

Serves: 6 Carbs: 27g Sugars: 13g Calories: 139

What you will need:

½ cup baking Splenda

1 /3 cup cocoa powder

1 teaspoon baking soda

1 teaspoon baking powder

2 tablespoons coconut oil

1 egg

Splash of vanilla

1 teaspoon molasses

1 tablespoon melted butter

½ cup nonfat milk

Directions:

Preheat oven to 350 degrees.

In one glass, oven safe dish, combine the dry ingredients, then add in the wet ingredients, one at a time.

Mix well, then place in the oven (use the same bowl as you did for mixeing). Of course you can change baking dishes if you like, but who doesn't want to save cleaning more dishes?

Bake for 20-30 minutes, testing with a butter knife before you take it out of the oven.

Let stand a few minutes, then enjoy!

Sparkling Spritzers

Serves: 1 Carbs: 10g Sugars: 13g Calories: 20

What you will need:

1 glass soda water

½ cup blueberries

Splash of pineapple juice

Ice

Directions:

Add the fruit to the soda water, then finish with the ice. Perfectly refreshing after dinner indulgence!

Lovely Lemon Cookies

Serves: 24 Carbs: 11g Sugars: 5g Calories: 60

What you will need:

1 cup whole wheat pastry flour

1/3 cup cornstarch

Salt

1/3 cup Splenda

2 tablespoons coconut oil

1 egg

Splash of vanilla

Splash of lemon juice

1 teaspoon lemon flavoring extract

Directions:

Preheat oven to 350 degrees F.

In a mixing bowl. Combine the dry ingredients first, followed by the wet ingredients. Mix well, until you have a nice dough. It may be crumbly, and if so, add in another teaspoon of the coconut oil.

Form 2 inch balls and place on a cookie sheet, then flatten with the bottom of a coffee mug. Bake in the oven for 8-10 minutes until done.

Enjoy!

Chocolatey Butter Bites

Serves: 9 Carbs: 9g Sugars: 10g Calories: 60

What you will need:

1 dark chocolate bar

½ tablespoon almond butter

Directions:

Break the chocolate bar into 9 pieces, then spread the almond butter evenly across each one.

Enjoy!

Frozen Pudding Cakes

Serves: 1 Carbs: 21g Sugars: 14g Calories: 79

What you will need:

¼ cup chocolate chips

1 graham cracker

Directions:

Melt the chocolate chips in a pan on the stove, then break your graham cracker in half. Spread the chocolate on the graham cracker, then close with the other side. Place in the freezer for a few hours, then enjoy.

Mini Cheesecakes

Serves: 1 Carbs: 17g Sugars: 1og Calories: 88

What you will need:

1 graham cracker

2 tablespoons cream cheese

2 large strawberries

Directions:

Slice the strawberries and soften the cream cheese. Combine the two then spread on the graham cracker. Enjoy!

Happy Ice Cream

Serves: 1 Carbs: 45g Sugars: 25g Calories: 201

What you will need:

1 packet Splenda

2 bananas

Splash of vanilla

Directions:

Freeze the bananas at least 4 hours, but the longer the better. Once your bananas are frozen, remove from the freezer and blend in your blender with a splash of vanilla.

Mix in the packet of Splenda, and enjoy!

Apple Cider Bites

Serves: 1 Carbs: 22 Sugars: 19 Calories: 95

What you will need:

1 apple

1 packet Splenda

Cinnamon

Nutmeg

Directions:

Slice your apple, and blend the spices and Splenda in another dish. Dip your apple in water, then blot it so it's not dripping wet, but not dry, either. Roll the apple in the spices, then set aside.

Once you have coated all of your apples, sit back and enjoy!

Whiteout Cake

Serves: 8 Carbs: 17g Sugars: 13g Calories: 147

What you will need:

1 cup whole wheat pastry flour

½ cup Splenda for baking

2 egg whites

1 tablespoon coconut oil

1 teaspoon baking soda

2 tablespoons vanilla

Salt

Directions:

Preheat your oven to 350 degrees F.

In a mixing bowl, combine all dry ingredients first, then add in the wet. Mix well. If the batter is too dry, add in a splash of milk or water.

Transfer to a greased baking dish, then place in the oven and bake for 30-40 minutes.

Test with a butter knife before removing from oven.

Enjoy!

White Chocolate Delight

Serves: 1 Carbs: 19g Sugars: 12g Calories: 101

What you will need:

1 graham cracker

1 ounce white chocolate chips

Directions:

Melt the white chips in a pan on the stove, and break the graham cracker into fourths. Dip the graham crackers into the chocolate chips, then let set up.

Enjoy!

Minty Madness

Serves: 1 Carbs: 24 Sugars: 12 Calories: 122

What you will need:

1 banana

¼ cup chocolate chips

¼ cup mint chips

Directions:

Melt the chocolate chips and mint chips in a pan on the stove. Dip the banana into the chocolate chips and let set up. Then dip in mint chips. Let set up once more, and enjoy!

Greek Grape Salad

Serves: 1 Carbs: 32 Sugars: 23g Calories: 112

What you will need:

1 cup grapes

½ cup plain low-fat Greek yogurt

Splash of vanilla

Packet of Splenda

Directions:

Combine the Splenda, vanilla and yogurt in a dish, then coat the grapes. Let chill in your fridge for a few hours, and enjoy!

Spectacular Chocolate Pudding

Serves: 1 Carbs: 8g Sugars: 10g Calories: 146

What you will need:

½ cup almond milk

Splash of vanilla

1/3 cup cocoa powder

2 packets Splenda

1 teaspoon xylitol

Directions:

Blend all ingredients in your blender until there are no lumps or clumps anywhere. Pour in a dessert cup in your fridge and let sit for a few hours. Enjoy.

Popcorn Delight

Serves: 1 Carbs: 26g Sugars: 5g Calories: 126

What you will need:

1 ounce popcorn

1 tablespoon dark chocolate chips

Directions:

Melt the chocolate in a pan on the stove, and drizzle over your popcorn. Lay out the popcorn so you can get an even coating, and let set up for a few minutes before you enjoy.

Iced Coffee for a King

Serves: 1 Carbs: 13g Sugars: 12g Calories: 66

What you will need:

1 *cup coffee*

1 ounce dark chocolate chips

1/3 cup vanilla almond milk

1 packet Splenda

Directions:

Melt the chocolate chips on the stove, and drizzle in your cup first. Carefully pour the coffee over the top, add in the almond milk next, then the Splenda.

Top with ice, and enjoy!

Fudge for All

Serves: 8 Carbs: 4g Sugars: Calories: 156

What you will need:

½ cup cocoa powder

1 cup unsweetened chocolate chips

2 packets Splenda

¼ cup vanilla almond milk

Directions:

Melt the chocolate chips and combine the rest of the ingredients into the pan. Transfer to a smaller pan and let set up for a couple hours to overnight.

Cut into small squares, and enjoy!

Chapter 8

The Fact of the Matter

"The fewer the facts, the stronger the opinion"

~Arnold H. Glasow

Chances are, if you have diabetes, you have at some point searched the internet for answers on whether or not you can cure or reverse your condition. You didn't need facts; you needed an answer.

You have a disease you don't want to have, and you want to get rid of it. It makes sense that you'd take to the internet. Of course, you found story after story of how people have effectively cured their diabetes with this little trick, or by doing that little thing.

All seemed lost until they did this one little thing you can pay to learn. Or, they tried and they tried until they found this one secret that no one else knew, and if you pay them, you can know it and get rid of your diabetes.

See the pattern?

If you take to the internet for answers, you are going to be told to pay to get the answer you want to hear, but you won't ever actually find any solid proofs or fact behind what is being said. You'll go on some wild goose chase to find the answers you want, but you will never be given the answers you need.

Which is what brings us to this chapter. I have given you things that will help your life as a whole, but I don't want to leave you hanging. I want to address the fact and the fiction once more, and take a serious and genuine look at how plausible it is for you to kick your diabetes once and for all.

Before we begin, I want to encourage you to face this chapter with an open mind. You might get exactly the answer you wanted, or you might get the exact opposite answer from the one you thought you needed.

Either way, you need to take the information that is given here and learn from it. This is all based on facts, not opinions, to learn from the facts and enrich your life, don't fight them and wish you could make things a certain way simply because some random person on the internet said it was so.

I am first going to address the question that is on the front of everyone's mind: Can you get rid of your diabetes through diet and exercise?

The answer for this is both simple and complex, all at the same time. The short answer is no, you can't completely cure yourself of diabetes through diet and exercise alone.

But again, that is just the short answer. You may know someone personally who was overweight and were no longer having diabetic blood results by losing the weight; you may have documented proof of someone who says that you can, and they may have documented proof of people who did.

But, remember the cancer analogy I used earlier? It applies once again here. You might know someone who was cured of cancer through chemotherapy, but you might know another person who goes to chemotherapy every day and discovers their cancer is worse every time they go in for an official test.

While I wish I could tell you that diet and exercise are a proven way to cure your diabetes, the fact of the matter is that they are not.

Now, this is no reason to give up or be discouraged in any way. While diet and exercise may not cure your diabetes, you are going to find that they do wonders to help manage your condition.

You may still have diabetes, but maybe you aren't going to have to take your pills. Perhaps you aren't going to feel so sick, and you are going to see the positive effects diet and exercise bring to your day. This in itself is enough reason to make diet and exercise a part of your daily routine, but it's not enough to say that you will for sure cure your diabetes through diet and exercise.

Now, with this all in mind, what are the statistics exactly? You have no doubt heard all these stories of people how have reversed their diabetes with diet and exercise, but what does that actually look like when it is put down on paper?

Before we get into the actual numbers, it's important to clear something up. First of all, when you have diabetes, you have something that is "chronic" — it's ongoing. Another aspect of the disease is that it is "progressive", which means it could get worse.

When you are diagnosed with diabetes, you are given medication to manage this illness. You are then prescribed to take the medication at various intervals for what is basically the rest of your life.

Now, when it comes to managing the illness as well as reversing the illness, you are met with a new set of statistics. Many, many people have been able to stop the progression of the disease through diet and exercise, and many, many people have been able to get off of their medication through diet and exercise.

When you read of those people who have been able to "reverse" their diabetes through diet and exercise, you are really looking at a lot of people who were able to get off their medication through diet and exercise. Don't misunderstand, there is a lot to be said for someone who is able to get off of their medication through diet and exercise, but that is not the same thing as someone who has never had the disease in the first place, or who is "cured."

Many times when you read of someone who has reversed their diabetes, you are reading of people who have gotten off their medication. Now, I am not saying they haven't done an incredible thing; what I am saying is that when it comes down to it, you need to focus on what you are doing with your medication rather than the disease itself.

While you may be feeling mixed emotions with this information, it's almost certain you are wondering what your chances are of reversing the illness in your own life.

The good news is that your chances are really, really good.

As it currently stands, the statistics point to being 1 in between 2 and 3 people being able to get off their medication through diet and exercise. That is nearly a 50% chance for you to do the same, which is really good as far as illness and medication go.

Even those who were not able to get off of their medication altogether saw an improvement in their daily living, were able to cut back on the dosage as well as the frequency they needed to take the medication and saw greater improvements in their number charts when they were at the doctor.

You see, when it comes down to reversing your diabetes, you can't focus solely on getting rid of the disease overall. It's about improving your quality of life. If you were to dedicate yourself to diet and exercise, and do everything within your power to follow all of the rules when it comes to diabetic living, you still may or may not get off your medication at the end of the day.

But, even if you don't, this doesn't mean that you should give up.

Let me clarify: *You decide you are going to do everything you can to reverse your diabetes and get off your medication. You are aware of the fact you may not cure yourself of the illness, but you do want to get off your medication.*

So what do you do?

You follow all the rules religiously. You do everything you are supposed to do, and you do nothing that you aren't. You follow each and every guideline to the letter, and you go above and beyond in the points you can. At the end of the day, you have done every single things possible to reverser your diabetes and get off your medication.

So, you go to the doctor full of high hopes. You are sure he's going to tell you that you can get off your medication. But instead, he tells you that while things are looking great and he's thrilled, he's going to keep you on your medication.

Now, to anyone who has been doing their absolute best to get off their medication, this is going to be very disheartening news. They tried and they tried, so what's the issue?

Well, the issue is the facts, and the fact of the matter is that you may not be able to get off your medication, even if you do everything as you should.

As we saw with the statistics, it's about 1 in 2 people who are able to get off their meds, and that's focusing on people who are doing everything they can to do it. I don't want to discourage you. In fact, I want to do everything I can to get you to see how much you can improve your life through diet and exercise, but I also want you to be prepared.

If you discover that you can't get off your medication, don't give up. The good you are doing for your health far exceeds what you would be like if you were on medication alone. Let the statistics be the statistics, and you do what is best for your health.

You never know when a cure is going to be created, and you want to be as close to diabetes free as you can be if that were to ever happen.

Chapter Takeaways

1. It's important to not take the internet at its word when you are looking for answers about your diabetes.

2. When people say they have reversed their diabetes, many are referring to getting off their medication, not being free of the illness altogether.

3. The fact is that you have about a 50/50 chance when it comes to reversing your own diabetes.

4. You can do everything within your power to reverse your diabetes and may still have to take your medication.

5. You can stop the progression of diabetes through diet and exercise, and if you have the goal of treating your diabetes without medication, you should focus on stopping it from progressing as much as you worry about reversing what has already been done.

Chapter 9

Life With Diabetes

"The life you have left is a gift, so cherish it and appreciate it to the fullest.

Do what matters, starting now."

- Kushondwizdom

Though it is extremely unfortunate, many people "cease to live" when they find out they have a disease of some kind. Sometimes that disease is something that really is crippling and mind blowing, but sometimes, it can be fully managed under the right conditions and with the right techniques.

I don't want you to be one of those people who allows a setback such as this to ruin their lives. It doesn't matter how old you are when you find out you have this illness; what matters is what you do after you discover the fact.

Many people just curl up and hide within themselves, others try to blame all their problems on the fact they have a disease. But others… the ones who truly go on to enjoy the life they still have, learn how to manage and cope with the disease, in spite of the hardships it may or may not push on their daily lives.

With this chapter, I want to show you what a normal life with diabetes looks like. I hope it encourages you to get out there and rekindle the things you used to enjoy doing, and perhaps even get out there and try a few new things. When it comes to diabetes, you really can live the life you want to live. You just have to take a few extra steps to be able to do it.

Typical day in the life of a person with diabetes:

Start your day with breakfast: one from the recipes earlier in the book would be a great start.

Walk for 10 minutes (or do jumping hacks, jogging, or anything to get your heart rate up).

Go about your morning, and have a healthy mid-morning snack to balance your blood sugar and hormones.

Lunch on time: again, one from earlier in this book is an excellent choice.

Walk for 10 more minutes (or again, do the exercise you prefer. This can be knee lifts, 10 minutes of active yoga, walking up and down stairs, or just walking).

Go about your afternoon, and don't forget your afternoon snack.

Check your insulin level at some point as well. This can be the same time every day, or this can be whenever you are feeling it, just make sure it gets done. Your doctor will have told you when you need to check it.

Dinner: You have from the recipes I have provided in this book, you have your pick of the crop. And, of course, the same goes for dessert.

Enjoy both guilt-free, then go on to do 10 more minutes of deliberate activity. This can be walking, jogging, walking up and down stairs, weight training, or anything that you enjoy doing - thirty minutes of activity a day is recommended, and by the end of this session you've reached that goal.

Go to bed, at the same time as last night if possible. Being timely and having a routine helps regulate your body's hormones and sugar processing.

And that's it. As you can see, you can do anything you normally do in a day, regardless of the job you work, the hobbies you have, of the schedule your day requires.

All you have to do is eat healthy foods regularly and exercise for 3o minutes a day, trying to break it up through the day so it's not too much at any one time.

Here are easy exercises you can do and they are fairly low-cost or free. They are effective, get your heart rate up (which is what you want) and they can fit into only 10 minutes at a time.

Choose walking, jogging, running, interval training, yoga, pilates, weight training or swimming. For some of the "class" type of exercises, go to your local library and pick up a DVD that you can use for several weeks for free - and the great part is, you can vary the types as often as you want for free. No regret that you purchased an expensive course that you hate - you can just go (maybe even walk) to the library and get a different one!

You get the idea. Basically anything that gets your heart rate up for at least 10 minutes at a time and anything you enjoy doing. If you don't see anything on this list you like, then find something you *do* enjoy.

There's bound to be something easy that gets the job done, and you are going to like it. Trust me, while exercise is a difficult hobby to break into, it's well worth the effort when you see the weight start to come off and your number chart start to stabilize.

Another "s" word for diabetics is socialize. For people with diabetes, it can be hard to know how to socialize, especially if you don't want to share with others the fact you have diabetes. First of all, diabetes should not make you feel ashamed; many, many people have it. But, there are still plenty of people who would rather keep the information to themselves, which is absolutely fine.

This does, however, make it difficult for when you are invited to parties, as there may not be things on the menu that you can have. If you are in this situation, you can take it on a case by case basis.

Either tell the host or hostess your preferences or eat beforehand so you can forego any treats at the party while still enjoying interacting with people. This may be difficult if you are going to a friend's house for dinner, and that may be a time when you have to offer one of the recipes I have provided earlier in this book.

As a general rule of thumb, however, you are going to be just fine. Though this may feel awkward at first, it's not going to be long before you settle into this as a way of life, and doing it will become second nature.

I find it's always easier to let a few people know what's happening, especially if you are going to be in a large group. But again, having diabetes is a personal thing, and whether you want someone else to know about it or not is also personal. Do what you want, what feels best and adjust your own actions accordingly.

Everyone wants to live a normal life, and if you have learned anything with this book, it's that you can live the normal life you want to live, even with diabetes. My dream for you is to settle into such a routine that you don't even realize you have the disease any longer. But doing that is going to require some effort on your part.

Part of this effort is going to be scoping out restaurants you can frequent, and keeping that mental list in mind for when you are going out with friends. Obviously, you are going to still date, even if you are married or partnered, you and your significant other will want to go out... which means you need to have specific places in mind to go.

No one wants to get stuck in a rut, and no one wants to only have a few options of places they can go. When it comes to having diabetes, eating out is going to require you to get creative, but don't worry, with a little bit of research, you can learn exactly what you can have at a variety of restaurants and where you can go that allows you to have virtually everything.

To do this, go online and read the menus. They tend to be complete, giving the nutrition information right along with the name of the food and the calories within the food. If you do some research in advance, all you have to do is decide where you go based on what you want to eat.

With practice, this is going to become so easy no one is even going to realize that you were insistent on the restaurant of choice, or that you already knew what you were going to get when you got there.

If you are still on the typical dating scene, you can easily get around this by suggesting to your date where you want to go when you ask her out. Or, when *you* are asked out, you can do the same thing… that is, suggest a restaurant to go or list the foods you like and you know are good for you,

As I said, with practice, you can do this so casually no one is going to realize that's what you really did.

Chapter Takeaways

1. Living a life with diabetes doesn't have to be remarkably different than living a normal life, you just have to take extra steps to make it happen.

2. It doesn't matter the kind of exercise you choose to do as long as you are going to stick with it, and as long as it gets your heart rate up (and keeps it there).

3. Prepare for dinner parties and social gatherings in advance, especially if you choose to keep your diabetes to yourself.

4. Do your research about the restaurants in your area and learn what foods you can have and where you can eat without worry.

5. Practice being natural about the foods you can eat and where you want to go to eat out… this is going to take the pressure off when you are invited out to dinner or when you want to meet friends.

One Last Thought

A diabetes diagnosis can be shocking, and will change your life. But, as you saw with this book, it doesn't have to have the shattering impact on your life that you initially think it's going to have.

Though it can be hard to accept the fact you have a chronic disease, you don't have to let it have any crippling effect on your life. With the right knowledge, the right information, and the right use of that information, you can live the same quality of life you lived before, only better.

I hope you take the information in this book and apply it to your day, and realize just how much your life can stay the same. It's going to take some practice to learn your new schedule, but with determination and dedication, you will pick it up quickly.

With the recipes you find in this book, you have nearly a month's worth of breakfasts, lunches and dinners all at your fingertips. To make it even better, you don't have to stress over the calories, carbs or sugar content in any one of them.

With these recipes, you can rest assured you have an entire list of food that is perfectly safe for you to have, but also up to your new health standards.

Now, it doesn't matter what's going on or if you suddenly have a surprise guest for dinner. If you know you have delicious recipes on hand, you can make any one of them at any time you need to take to a potluck or to have a house party.

And, to make things even better, I have given you the chance to make and bring desserts to any event. Events are going to be stress free and easy when you have a whole list of recipes!

Practice with each one until you find your favorites, and feel free to modify and change them to be exactly what you want them to be. When you know what you're doing because you are starting in the right spot, you have the freedom to do whatever you want when you want, just like you did before you had to pay attention to what you eat.

In addition to enjoying your freedom of food, don't forget to keep an eye on your charts. No matter how long you have diabetes, you will always need to keep an eye on your blood sugar level, your blood pressure and your weight. Of course, through proper diet and exercise, these things will all be easy to manage through your lifestyle alone.

But, that doesn't mean you can forget about the numbers. Keeping an eye on your range and specifics is going to allow you to track patterns and variations. This is going to give you better insight on how you are affected by certain foods and exercises, as well as how you good you feel in a certain range.

The more of a handle you have on your diabetes, the less you will have to worry about these numbers, but now you know that you aren't ever going to reach a point where you can forget about the chart altogether.

Understand that life is ever growing and changing, and the fact you have diabetes is just another step along the way.

Many people get diagnosed, then spend their entire life revolving their choices around their diabetes. While you will always have to keep the fact you have diabetes in the back of your mind, and many choices you make are going to be in regards to your condition, you don't have to let this rule your life.

With a healthy diet plan and an exercise regimen you enjoy, this is going to be just another thing in your day.

Life is full of ups and downs, and the good times and bad. Diabetes is one of those things that happens, but can be overcome. Don't be one of those people who lets this control their lives. Don't be one of those people who depends on medication to take care of everything.

Be one of those people who takes life by the horns and gets things done. Be an achiever. Be a winner.

Could You Help?

I'd love to hear your feedback about my book. In the world of publishing, there are few things more valuable than honest reviews from a wide variety of readers.

Your review will help other readers find out if my book is for them. It will also help me reach more readers by increasing the visibility of this book and helps see what other topics could inspire you to do better things.

Printed in Poland
by Amazon Fulfillment
Poland Sp. z o.o., Wrocław